How to Get Rid of Insomnia Naturally

By M. Usman

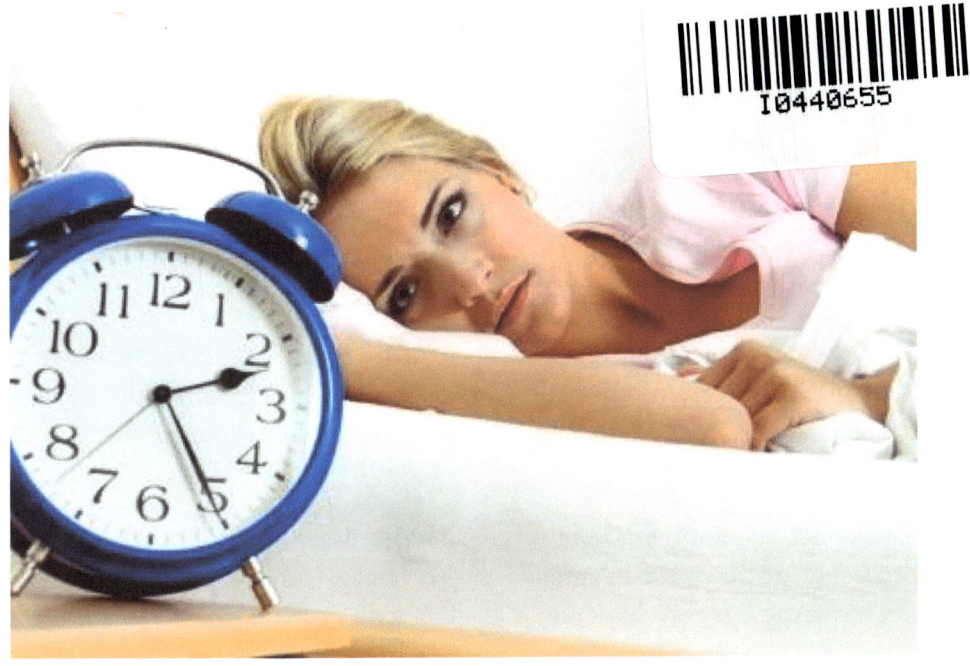

Health Learning Series

Mendon Cottage Books

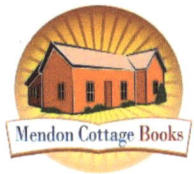

JD-Biz Publishing

Disclaimer

The information is this book is provided for informational purposes only. It is not intended to be used and medical advice or a substitute for proper medical treatment by a qualified health care provider. The information is believed to be accurate as presented based on research by the author.

The contents have not been evaluated by the U.S. Food and Drug Administration or any other Government or Health Organization and the contents in this book are not to be used to treat cure or prevent disease or mental illness.

The author or publisher is not responsible for the use or safety of any diet, procedure or treatment mentioned in this book. The author or publisher is not responsible for errors or omissions that may exist.

Warning

The Book is for informational purposes only and before taking on any diet, treatment or medical procedure it is recommended to consult with your primary care provider.

Our books are available at

1. Amazon.com

2. Barnes and Noble

3. Itunes

4. Kobo

5. Smashwords

6. Google Play Books

Table of Contents

Preface..*6*

Getting Started..*7*

Chapter # 1: Introduction..7

Chapter # 2: Types of Insomnia....................................9

Classification based on the underlying cause:..................9

Classification according to frequency: 10

Other types: 11

Insomnia due to specific lifestyle:.................................12

Chapter # 3: Complications 13

Chapter # 4: Signs & Symptoms 14

Chapter # 5: Optimum duration of Sleep......................16

Understanding Insomnia....................................... *17*

Chapter # 6: Causes of Insomnia..................................17

Stress: 17

Depression:...17

Physical Condition: 17

Drug and Substance abuse: 18

Poor Sleeping Habits:...18

Learned Insomnia:..18

Medication: 19

Overeating:...19

Chapter # 7: Who gets insomnia?..................................21

Chapter # 8: Insomnia and Aging..................................23

Cures to Insomnia... *25*

Chapter # 9: Overview...25

Chapter # 10: Overcome Stress 26

Exercise: 26

Brain training games: 28

Be a part of society: 28

Have healthier relationships: 28

Enjoy free time: 29

Avoid anger: 29

Do not overburden yourself: 29

Chapter # 11: Lifestyle change 30

Leave smoking behind: 30

Cut down on Alcohol: 31

Physical activity: 31

Change your Environment: 31

Reading: 32

Music: 32

Meals: 33

Avoid long naps: 33

Chapter # 12: Natural Foods 34

Almonds: 34

Tea: 34

Miso Soup: 34

Banana: 35

Dairy: 35

Oatmeal: 35

Full-boiled egg: 35

Immature soybeans: 36

Cherries: 36

Chapter # 13: Relaxing the Mind 37

Conclusion.. *40*

References *41*

Author Bio... *42*

Publisher *53*

Preface

Insomnia- not an uncommon word and is experienced by many, some go through it frequently, while others quite rarely. But what is insomnia exactly? Is it when you're not able to sleep? Yes, maybe, but for how long? And how many times must you experience sleeping troubles before you think you have insomnia?

The medical community defines insomnia as the inability to attain sleep. Insomnia isn't a disease, rather, it is categorized as a 'sleeping disorder'; when a patient complains of facing troubles in getting proper sleep, or is experiencing 'sleeplessness'. To put it simply, there are two aspects of this disorder- either difficulty when falling asleep, or inability to stay asleep for an appropriate period of time.

One cannot diagnose insomnia all by him/herself; it is clinically predicted by several factors. Moreover, the condition may either prevail in its simple isolated form, or may be complicated by the presence of other diseases or predisposing factors.

Don't worry as each of your questions will be answered! Everything you need to know about insomnia is in this book, its signs, its cures, its causes; simply everything. So take a load off and start reading!

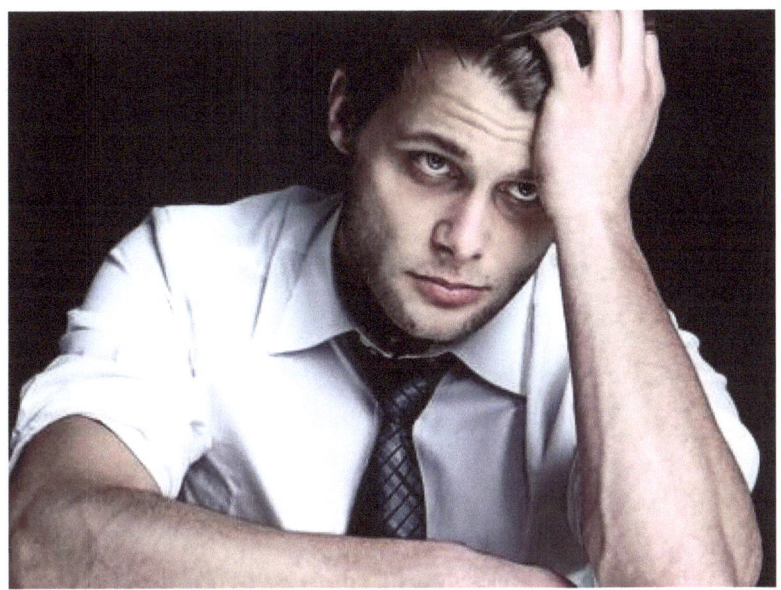

Getting Started

Chapter # 1: Introduction

Many amongst us experience insomnia at some points in our lives, though we may not be always aware of the root cause.

Have you ever gone through a situation when you're lying on your bed for more than an hour and there isn't any hint of sleep? And to deliberately make yourself fall asleep, you grab a book and start reading it, count on fingers, or even follow that really old method of counting imaginary sheep, but still you are wide awake.

This inability to fall asleep is what is termed as 'insomnia' by medical experts.

That's not all. Has there been a time when you are woken up suddenly, from sleep at various irregular intervals, and it continues to happen all night long? This kind of condition in which one faces a disturbed sleep all night long can also be classified as insomnia.

Generally, insomnia patients tend to respond positively to queries such as, 'Do you think you have difficulties in attaining sleep?' or, 'Do you think you are unable to sleep peacefully and keep waking up many times.'

Chapter # 2: Types of Insomnia

Although it appears to be a simple medical condition, but insomnia is widely categorized into various types, with almost each category varying greatly. Some medical experts have classified it according to its prime cause, while others have focused more upon the pattern which the disorder tends to follow. The following are the descriptions of each of the classifications.

Classification based on the underlying cause:

According to this classification, insomnia is divided into two types; Primary and Secondary:

- **Primary insomnia:** When insomnia occurs without the presence of any disease; meaning, when the sleeping disorder is not attributed to any other disease or ailment, it is then called as primary insomnia.

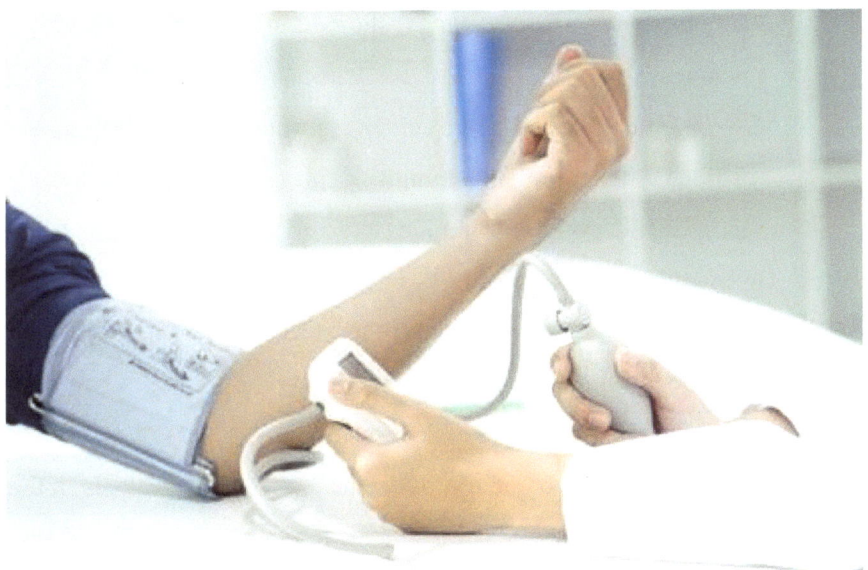

- **Secondary insomnia:** Insomnia is said to be secondary when it occurs due to any prevailing disease; its intensity depends upon the type of disease. Furthermore, disorders that are related to psychology can also produce insomnia. For instance, patients diagnosed with depression often complain of having a disturbed sleep. Other than psychological ailments, other diseases that produce secondary insomnia include arthritis, asthma, central sleep apnea, etc.

Classification according to frequency:

According to the frequency of its occurrence and the amount of time it prevails, the sleeping disorder can be grouped as follows:

- **Acute insomnia:** When disturbances with attaining sleep or staying asleep last less than a month, the condition is called, acute insomnia. Usually attributed to stress such as a hectic routine, exams, etc. it is also known as 'short-term' or 'stress related' insomnia.

- **Chronic insomnia:** Unlike acute insomnia, chronic sleeping disorder lasts more than a month. It can either be primary or secondary. Chronic insomnia casts many negative impacts on an individual's overall health, as well as disturbs his psychology. But these effects may be related to other diseases, the ones which produce insomnia.

- **Transient insomnia:** Transient insomnia lasts less than a week. It is usually triggered due to minor reasons, such as changes in the usual timings of one's sleep, changes in the environment of sleep like travelling to another part of the world.

Other types:

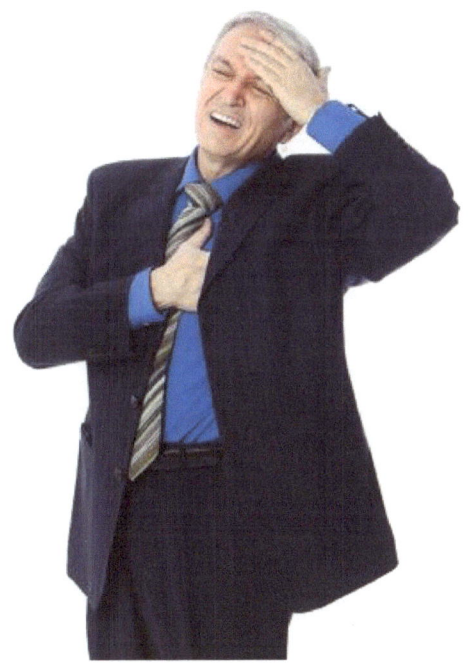

- **Psychophysiological insomnia:** This kind of sleeplessness occurs due to excessive worrying regarding one's sleep. Such individuals worry too much about their poor sleep problem, as well as its effects on their routine the next day; basically, it's like being depressed specifically about your sleep.
- **Paradoxical insomnia:** Patients with paradoxical insomnia complain of being deprived of sleep or having little for a night or more than that.

Insomnia due to specific lifestyle:

Several external factors have been discovered that highly affect one's sleep. Substance abuse is the most common trigger to insomnia. People who consume high amounts of caffeine are also known to complain of having problems related to their sleep. Improper habits throughout the day such as lack of physical activities and improper diet and meal timings are yet another cause.

Chapter # 3: Complications

Sleep deserves the same amount of attention as a healthy diet or physical fitness. Whatever might be the reason for your insomnia; it can affect you mentally as well as physically. The side-effects of insomnia include:

- Lower performance at work.
- Lowered thinking skills.
- Higher risk of accidents.
- Slowed Reaction time.
- Obesity.
- Immaturity in the immune system.
- Increased risk of long term diseases.
- Unsettled social life.

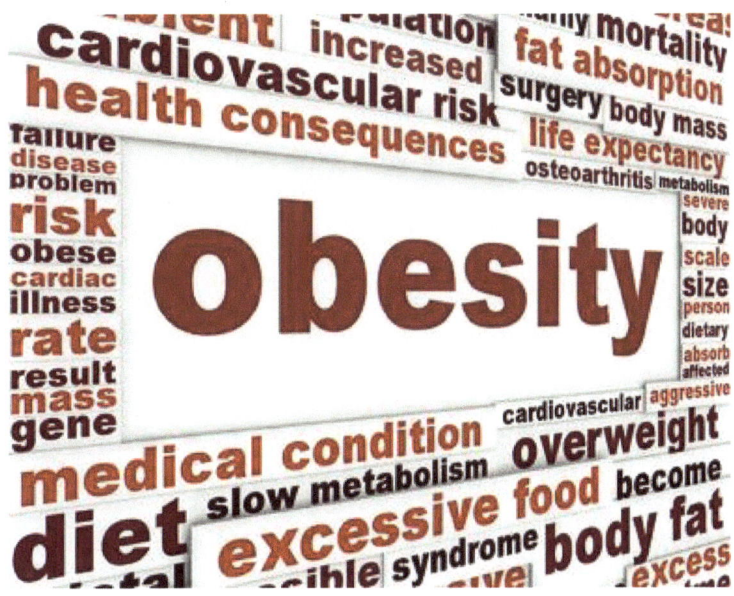

Chapter # 4: Signs & Symptoms

The one good news for people who suffer from insomnia is that, it is quite easy to diagnose insomnia personally. The list of symptoms of insomnia is quite comprehensive therefore; diagnosing insomnia is not a hefty job. The list is given below:

- Waking up in the middle of night.
- Waking up too early in the morning.
- Difficulty falling asleep at night.
- Feeling restless, even after a good night's sleep.
- Feeling lethargic and fatigued during the day.
- Feeling irritated on small issues.
- Feeling nauseated; loss of appetite.
- Under the effects of depression and anxiety.
- Difficulty in thinking and focusing on tasks.
- Increased mistakes or errors in work.
- Headaches.
- Being worried about sleep itself.

If you are still unsure, as to whether you have insomnia or not; ask yourself the following questions:

- ✓ Do you wake up during the night?
- ✓ Do you find it increasing hard to go to sleep after an unscheduled wake up?
- ✓ Do you avoid going to bed because you find it unable to catch a good night's sleep?
- ✓ Do you lie in bed, turning and tossing for hours?
- ✓ Do you wake up, all nauseated after sleeping?

✓ Does the problem occur, even though you have all the conditions for a good night's sleep?

If the answer to two or more than two of the questions given above is yes, then unfortunately you have insomnia.

Chapter # 5: Optimum duration of Sleep

Every person is different; many factors influence the "normal sleep time" including age, lifestyle, diet and environment. The following table will give you an idea of the amount of sleep you need based on your age.

Age	Sleep Time
Newborns (0-2 months)	12-18 hours
Infants (3-11 months)	14-15 hours
Toddlers (1-3 years)	12-14 hours
Preschoolers (3-5 years)	11-13 hours
School-age children (5-10 years)	10-11 hours
Teens (10-17 years)	8-9 hours
Adults (18 +)	7-9 hours

If you do not sleep according to the specifications in the table above, that might be another reason as to why you undergo insomnia.

Understanding Insomnia

Chapter # 6: Causes of Insomnia

Before moving forward to the cures of insomnia it is vital to understand the causes of insomnia. Insomnia may be caused by various, diverse things such as a stressful event, physical conditions, drug abuse.

Stress:

A lot of people complain about insomnia due to a stressful or traumatic event; the insomnia tends to continue even when the effects of stress/trauma have gone. The reason behind this is the mind learns to associate sleeping habits with being alert which makes you wake up at nights and prevents you from falling asleep. Worrying about work, health, money, a loved one, all add to factors that keep you awake.

Depression:

Depression may cause excess sleeping or under-privileged sleeping. This behavior of the body is due to chemical imbalances in the brain or worries that take up all your attention throughout the day. That is not all; if you get insomnia through depression; other mental disorders tends to follow.

Physical Condition:

Conditions like chronic pain, breathing difficulties or unitary problems can all increase the intensity of your insomnia. Specific medical conditions linked with insomnia include, arthritis, heart failure, cancer, lung disease, overactive thyroid stroke, Parkinson's and Alzheimer's disease. These conditions must be treated under the guidance of a health care provider, and if treated successfully can take a lot of load of your insomnia.

Drug and Substance abuse:

Coffee, cola, tea and other caffeine-induced drinks are known stimulants. Having these drinks late in the afternoon can keep you from sleeping at night. Nicotine is another stimulant that can cause insomnia. It is most commonly found in tobacco. Alcohol is a sedative that is ingested to help falling asleep; but the major side effect of alcohol is preventing deeper stages of sleep that results in unsatisfied feelings in the morning.

Poor Sleeping Habits:

Sleep is promoted by habits called sleep hygiene. Poor sleep hygiene means random sleeping times, stimulating activities before going to sleep, unhealthy environment and use of bed for activities other than sleeping

Learned Insomnia:

This is a very interesting yet true phenomenon; it occurs when you try to fall asleep and worry about not being able to do so. They spend hours wondering about this until they indulge themselves in other activities.

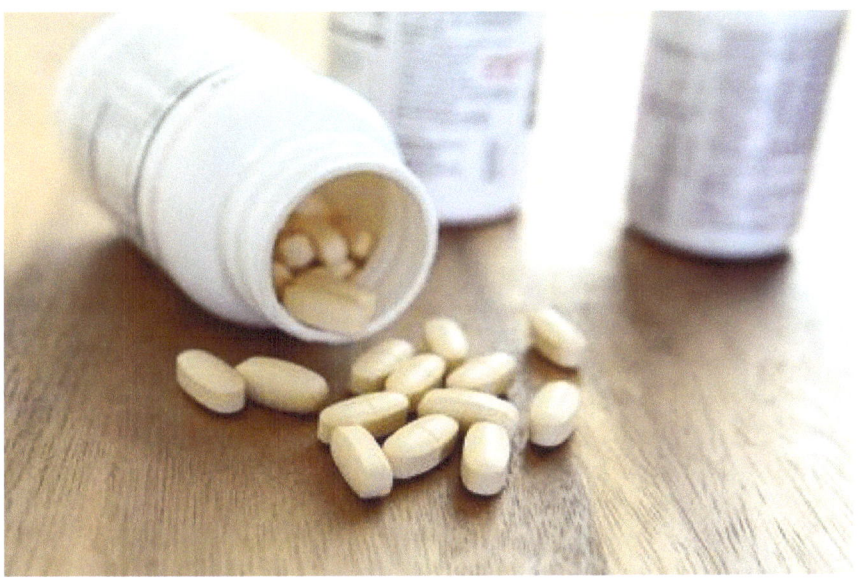

Medication:

Prescription drugs can also interfere with your sleep; drugs including anti-depressants, blood and heart medications, allergy medications and corticosteroids, all cause insomnia. Moreover, many OTC (over the counter) medications including pain killers, decongestants and gastric products also make you lethargic.

Overeating:

A little snack before bed time is alright but eating just for the sake of filling yourself is madness and results in feelings of physical displeasure. People experience inflammation from backflow of acid into the esophagus and other such conditions, all of which interfere with your sleep.

Chapter # 7: Who gets insomnia?

Even though anyone is prone to insomnia, some people have a greater chance of suffering from it. These can be categorized as:

- **Gender:**

  Women are more prone to develop insomnia. However, the level of disturbances with sleep is equal in both the genders. The reason behind this gender fact is that, the hormonal shifts during menstrual cycles, pregnancy and menopause casts effects on the sleep pattern, producing insomnia in some women.

- **Senior citizens:**

  An increased age also stands as a risk factor in some aged individuals. Age above sixty can make one prone to insomnia due to changes in the sleeping pattern.

- **Work shift changes:**

  Working in changing shifts can also produce insomnia. Night shift workers experience insomnia more as compared to those who work during the day time.

- **Too much of travelling:**
  This is yet another risk factor for insomnia. People who travel many times over different time zones tends to have a relatively messed up biological clock.

- **Unfavorable sleeping environment:**

  Those who sleep in an environment with several distractions, such as television, noise, too much light, etc. are very likely to experience insomnia.

- **Adolescents:**

  The reason behind this is quite clear; they have too much on their plates. People with jobs are not the only one who get stressed. Young adult students also suffer through periods of tensions due to exams, projects and relationships.

Chapter # 8: Insomnia and Aging

Insomnia becomes more serious with age. As you grow older the intensity of insomnia increase due to the following reasons:

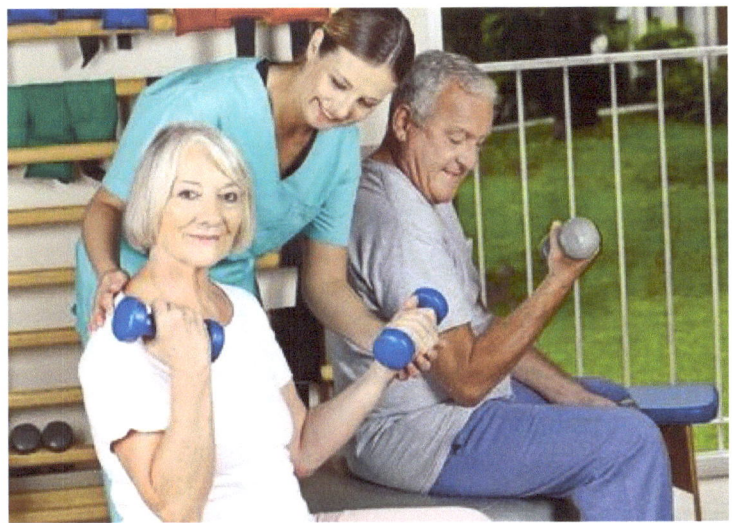

- A change in sleep patterns. As you age you will notice that the slightest changes in the environment like a little light or a sound would put you off. With age your internal clock changes; you get tired early, therefore, sleep early and hence wake up early. This can disrupt a person's whole lifestyle as not all elder people rest all day.
- A change in activity. Some senior citizen may have a retirement plan and get less physically active. Remember that activity promote a good night's sleep. Furthermore, elder people take naps during day time too; this disturbs their sleeping patterns and they suffer from insomnia.

- A change in health. Chronic pains such as arthritis and psychiatric disorders like depression can interfere with sleep. Older people also develop a larger prostate gland that causes the need to urinate more frequently which results in difficulty in sleeping.
- Increased use of medications. As older people have a greater chance of catching an ailment they also use a greater amount of medication. This also increases their chance of suffering from insomnia.

Cures to Insomnia

Chapter # 9: Overview

Once diagnosed with insomnia, your doctor shall prescribe you a list of medicines or maybe even advice you to visit the clinic for therapies, if needed.

But there is an alternative method as well. If you do not wish to solve your sleeping disorder through clinical means, you can work on them all by yourself, from the convenience of your home.

Such natural methods involve, changing your lifestyle habits, reducing stress, implementing certain activities in your schedule that would help you to sleep better, introducing various changes in your meals that can help your body correct its sleeping pattern, etc.

Natural methods for the treatment of insomnia are way too useful if the cause of your sleeping disorder is unknown. Correcting lifestyle pattern may turn out as a solution for your sleeping problem.

Although these natural methods can be followed by anyone, it is advised that you visit your health care provider; if your insomnia is dependent on a disease or disorder.

Chapter # 10: Overcome Stress

As discussed above, stress plays a great role in the disruption of your normal sleep cycle. Stress can be managed in many ways; following are some useful ways to put off stress.

Exercise:

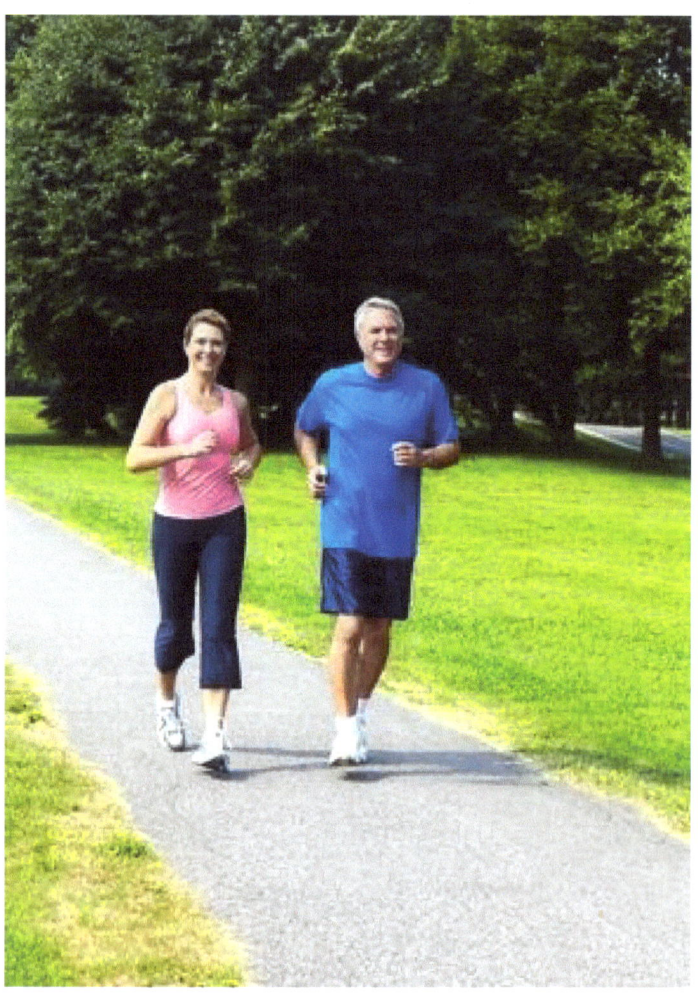

The most appropriate method to fight off stress is by exercising. In fact, one must exercise daily, whether they are stressed out or not. Through various research studies, it has been proved that, the things one practices when he/she is feeling normal are the things he/she is most likely to do when he/she is under the effects of stress. Hence, if you make yourself habitual to unhealthy habits in usual situations, your mind shall insist acting the same when it is stressed.

- Jog, walk or run along tracks for at least half an hour daily in the morning, in a fresh environment. It is preferable to go to parks for exercising where, in addition to exercising, you can also socialize.
- Swimming is also a great activity. It is an overall exercise package for both the mind and the body.
- Go for cycling. Try to find a partner and this will help you a lot.
- Gyms are also good venues to exercise and socialize at the same time. But, an open and natural environment is more preferable.
- Indulge in sporting activity. Become a member of sports club in your area or institute, or if you do not have time for that, go out in the evening with friends and play badminton, basketball, volley ball, or some other game.

The reason why exercise is so good at eliminating stress is because it stimulates the pumping of endorphins into the blood, which in turn, provide the body with pleasant feeling. It improves blood circulation to various parts of the body, enhancing their function, including the central nervous system. With a better functioning brain, your capability to fight off stress and to tackle problems efficiently increases. With the release of endorphins and an enhanced thinking system, your mood goes up automatically. A good mood means lesser stress.

If you keep up your exercising habits this way, you will bring your stress levels down and hence, experience a better sleep.

Brain training games:

Train your brain to tackle problems. Play interesting brain training games. If you love math, solve math problems regularly. Brain training games not only help your mind in increasing its efficiency, but it also diverts your attention from stress igniting tasks.

Fifteen minutes of a game or any other training activity is quite enough. But make sure that you do no indulge too much into it, so much so that you get addicted to it!

Be a part of society:

Every individual forms an integral part of the society. Prove your importance by becoming an active member. Help your society by any means that you find is convenient for you. Volunteer work can prove very helpful, both for you and for the society; it will show you that you are also a vital part of the society and alleviate stress.

All this helps you turn down stress in a way that it avoids you to indulge too much into your work. Moreover, it increases your knowledge and skills and makes you aware of problems with people greater than your own.

Have healthier relationships:

Avoid relationships that are temporary. Choose relationships that are going to last and will be worth something in the future. Additionally, try having strong bonds with your family as they are the closest thing to you. Share your issues with your closest friend or your partner; speak out your problems and seek for a solution from them when you unable to find one on your own.

Enjoy free time:

Free time or holidays are given to you for one reason only; to relax. So do not waste it by working or worrying about working. Instead, enjoy it by doing things you didn't have a chance to do till now but at the same time staying away from danger. Go out with friends on a road trip, host reunion parties, go hiking, skiing; the choices are unlimited.

Avoid anger:

Avoid getting angry too often; it brings out no good except stress. Regain control over your nerves and try to solve every problem logically. If you find it too hard to control your anger and are afraid that it might get physical, then leave the room/situation and take a deep breath, hold it in for a while, and then exhale.

Do not overburden yourself:

Work for the sake of work but do not let it interfere with your personal life. Do not overburden yourself and work according to your capacity, if you work keeps you up late at nights then it would only mess up with your body clock and after a few days, your insomnia will develop into chronic insomnia. Moreover, avoid work getting piled up at your desk; work with full concentration so you wouldn't have to face this problem.

Chapter # 11: Lifestyle change

Implementing, changing and omitting certain habits from your lifestyle can magically resolve you sleeping disorder. Little habits that might seem harmless in your perspective might be the cause of insomnia in your life.

Leave smoking behind:

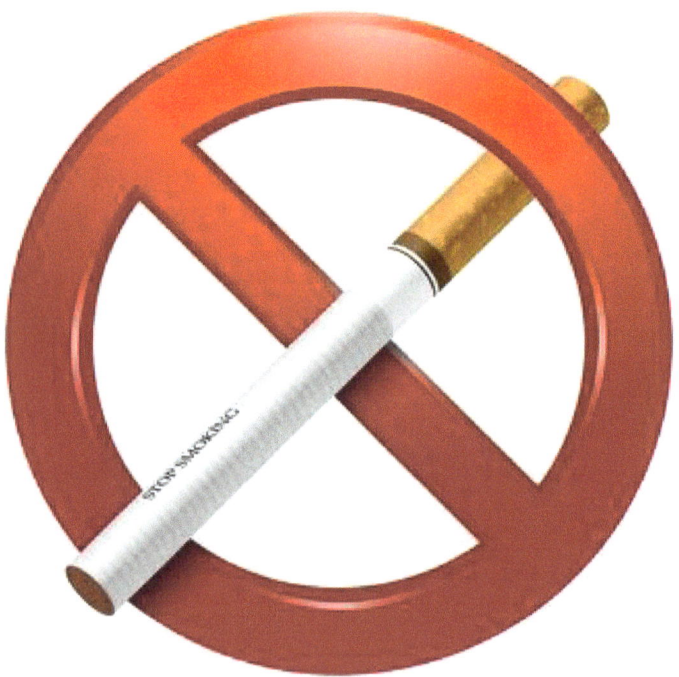

The negative impacts of smoking have been emphasized in the previous section. In a nutshell, besides deteriorating the lungs greatly, the ingredients of a cigarette arouse the central nervous system and in this way keep a person from sleeping.

No doubt that cutting down smoking altogether is a difficult goal so, try to reduce the amount of cigarettes you smoke a day; from half the amount you normally take a day to the amount you take a week. Fill the usual times with other foods or activities such as apples. In this way gradually decrease your intake and you will be able to find relief in your sleep.

Cut down on Alcohol:

Alcohol is another factor that is known to induce insomnia. Those who drink alcoholic beverages many times in a day are found to be complaining of sleeping troubles. So follow the same regimen as described with smoking; try your best to avoid drinking before you sleep as it is very damaging in the long run.

Physical activity:

Make sure that you perform adequate amounts of physical activity per day even if you don't have stress. A lazy lifestyle won't allow you to sleep properly either. If your body is completely utilized it would need sleep; this would help you sleep almost instantly, sometimes without the added hassle of reading books and watching TV.

Change your Environment:

Things like television, music players, and even your cell phone can act as distracting objects when you are trying to fall asleep. Your room should be dark and quite when you are ready to doze off. Additionally, the environment should remain quiet for the whole time as distractions in between your sleep.

- ✓ Use thick blinds and wear an eye mask if you are distracted by light at sunrise.
- ✓ Wear ear plugs if noise is not avoidable.
- ✓ A comfortable mattress, a pillow and enough sheets to cover you up.

Put away your cell phone or place it on silent mode so that, unnecessary stuff doesn't interfere with your snooze.

Also, make sure that you have completed all your important work before you are off to bed. Leaving something undone that would irritate you when you are trying to fall asleep would make you restless in bed all night.

Reading:

This is the oldest and by far the most widely effective remedy for falling asleep. Sufferers of insomnia can develop a habit of reading to go to sleep; it doesn't matter if the material is interesting or not. Just starting reading it and you'll fall asleep.

Music:

Some people find music as a way to attain peace of mind. If you do listen to music, choose soothing, low beat genres and not heavy metal and rock songs; this will help you quite a lot in falling asleep and keep all distracting noises outside.

*Keep the volume of your device below 75% to avoid any damage to your ears.

Meals:

Before sleeping, the body systems slow down its functions. Avoid eating very heavy meals for dinner and always take a walk before going to bed. This will help in putting you to sleep. Furthermore, eating late at night is also unfavorable for your body as it will make your digestive system work for hours and hence, that would ultimately interrupt your sleep.

Avoid long naps:

A little snooze in the afternoon hours is really good, it refreshes your mind. But don't fall asleep longer than 30 – 45 minutes as sleeping more than that can put off your night sleeping time.

Chapter # 12: Natural Foods

Over the counter medications are not the only things that can help you fall asleep. Eating the right foods before you hit the bed can help you too; the natural remedies are quite simple too. Here are some that would help you sleep properly.

Almonds:

Almonds are winners when it comes to putting you to sleep. They have magnesium, an element that promotes sleep and muscle relaxation. Furthermore, they have the benefit of supplying proteins that help maintain stable blood sugar during one's sleep. In simple words, it switches your body from alert adrenaline cycle to rest-and-digest cycle. So have at most a tablespoon of almond butter or an ounce of almonds to help you go to sleep.

Tea:

Don't worry it's not decaf! Yes, avoiding all caffeine products in the evening is the key to a good night's sleep but teas like chamomile tea and green tea can be very helpful. Green tea contains theanine that promotes sleep. One cup of tea before going to bed would be all that is required.

Miso Soup:

Everyone loves to have this comforting, Japanese soup at restaurants but keeping a few packs of instant soups, right in your home can help you if you have trouble falling asleep. Miso contains amino acids that boost the production of the natural hormone melatonin known for its induction of yawns in the body. Plus, it's great if you have a fever or a cold!

Banana:

Everyone knows that bananas are an excellent source of potassium but only few people know what potassium does. Potassium when combined with magnesium (which bananas also have) help to relax overstressed muscles. They contain a compound, tryptophan, which converts the brain's calming hormones to serotonin. Try the following tasty and simple bed time smoothie if you don't like raw bananas; blend one banana with a cup of milk (soy if you want). Add some ice and enjoy.

Dairy:

Milk, cheese and yogurt all have sleep-inducing effects. This is because they contain calcium which is an effective stress reluctant and stabilizer of nerve fibers. Thus, by reducing stress, dairy products can help you go to sleep.

Oatmeal:

Apart from being a healthy breakfast, oatmeal can also help you get more rest. It has all the vital nutrients, i.e. calcium, magnesium, silicon, potassium and phosphorus; plus it it's soft, soothing and easy to prepare. Prepare your oatmeal just as normal but replace sugar with fruit to avoid any anti-calming effect.

Full-boiled egg:

One of the reasons as to why you are unable to sleep at nights is because of low protein intake before bedtime. If this habit is combined with high-sugar carbs like cake then sleeping can become quite difficult. The problem with carbs is that they dip your blood sugar which causes you to wake up at late at night. So eat an egg with nuts, not to just fall asleep but to stay asleep.

Immature soybeans:

Care for a salty snack just before bed? Then turn to lightly salted edamame or soybeans. The natural estrogen-like products found in them can be very beneficial in controlling nighttime flashes that disturb your sleep. This easy recipe can give you both taste and comfort: Use a food processor to blend two cups of shelled and cooked edamame with a tablespoon salt, some drops of olive oil and a clove until smooth.

Cherries:

Another effective way to fall asleep is cherry juice. In a study conducted by researchers from the University of Pennsylvania, they found that cherries, especially tart cherries, boosted the body's stock of melatonin; this helped people in falling asleep. Sipping a glass of cherry juice or having a fresh, frozen serving before bedtime can help you with falling asleep.

Chapter # 13: Relaxing the Mind

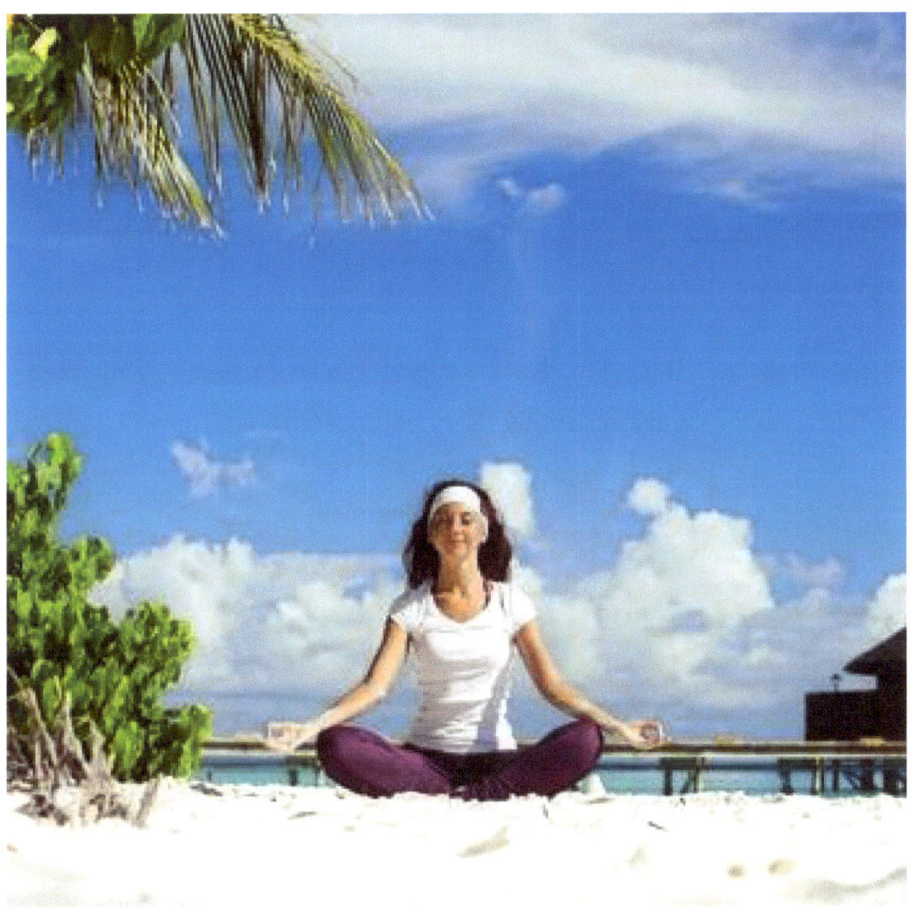

Step 1: Lie in a comfortable position in bed and take five deep breaths, using your nose for breathing in and your mouth for breathing out. As you breathe in, visualize your lungs getting filled with air and while you breathe out, replace that air with your thoughts of the day and imagine them leaving your body.

Step 2: Now check in with how you're feeling. Remember that you cannot rush through sleep in the same way that you cannot rush through relaxation so take your time and analyze every feeling that comes your way.

Step 3: Become aware of your physical surroundings, the points of contacts with the bed, your weight sinking in to the mattress. If there is a sound and it's out of your control; rather than resisting it, rest your attention on it. Keep your attention on the sound for about a minute before bringing your attention back to the body.

Step 4: Next, scan down your body and get a sense of how it actually feels, from head to toe gently, observing every point of tension. You will notice that the mind will be drawn to areas of pain and tightness. Nevertheless, focus on each area.

Step 5: Now go back to the activities of the day in a structured way. Start off by remembering the first thing you did in the morning to going to work. Notice as your mind plays a fast-forward of the day's events; still go through every activity in about three minutes until you're finally brought into the present moment.

Step 6: Now as you're back into the present moment, bring your attention to the body. Focus on your toes of either foot and imagine as if they're turning off. Repeat the words if it helps. It is as if you're giving your toes the permission to go offline and become unresponsive. Repeat this with the remaining part of the foot and slowly move up the leg. But before switching to the other leg, do notice if you feel different in the leg that has been "turned off"; any doubt in your mind as to whether this exercise is working will clear up now.

Step 7: Continue the exercise with the remaining parts of body up till your head. Take a moment to enjoy the tension-free sensation that goes through your body. Your mind is now free to wander as much as it wants, from one thought to another, until of course you go to sleep!

Conclusion

Insomnia may sound like a minor issue but those who suffer from it can do anything to get rid of it. This book explains that the take-the-pill treatment is not the only way to get rid of insomnia. Instead you can perform other activities to purge insomnia and its effects. This book will prove to be the ultimate guide on curing insomnia through natural means so flip it open and get ready to wave the sleepless nights goodbye.

References

http://www.fotolia.com/id/50889876

http://www.fotolia.com/id/47136007

http://www.fotolia.com/id/48701190

http://www.fotolia.com/id/45319152

http://www.fotolia.com/id/45257208

http://www.fotolia.com/id/48980656

http://www.fotolia.com/id/49218655

http://www.fotolia.com/id/39676947

http://www.fotolia.com/id/39332640

http://www.fotolia.com/id/46615428

http://www.fotolia.com/id/51931924

http://www.fotolia.com/id/51141099

Author Bio

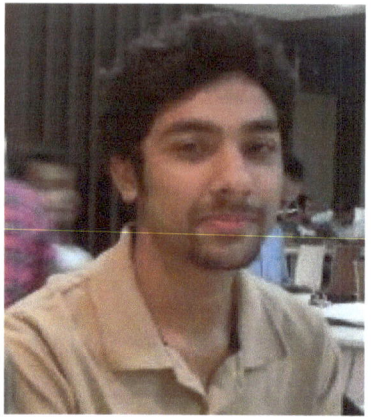

Muhammad Usman is a distinguished medical graduate of Allama iqbal medical college (AIMC). He is a professional writer who has been in the field for more than 4 years. During this time he has produced 10,000+ articles, blogs and eBooks on various niches related to diseases, health, fitness, nutrition and well-being. He is a regular contributor to several journals related to medicine and surgery. He is the editor of several journals and newspapers.

Check out some of the other JD-Biz Publishing books

Gardening Series on Amazon

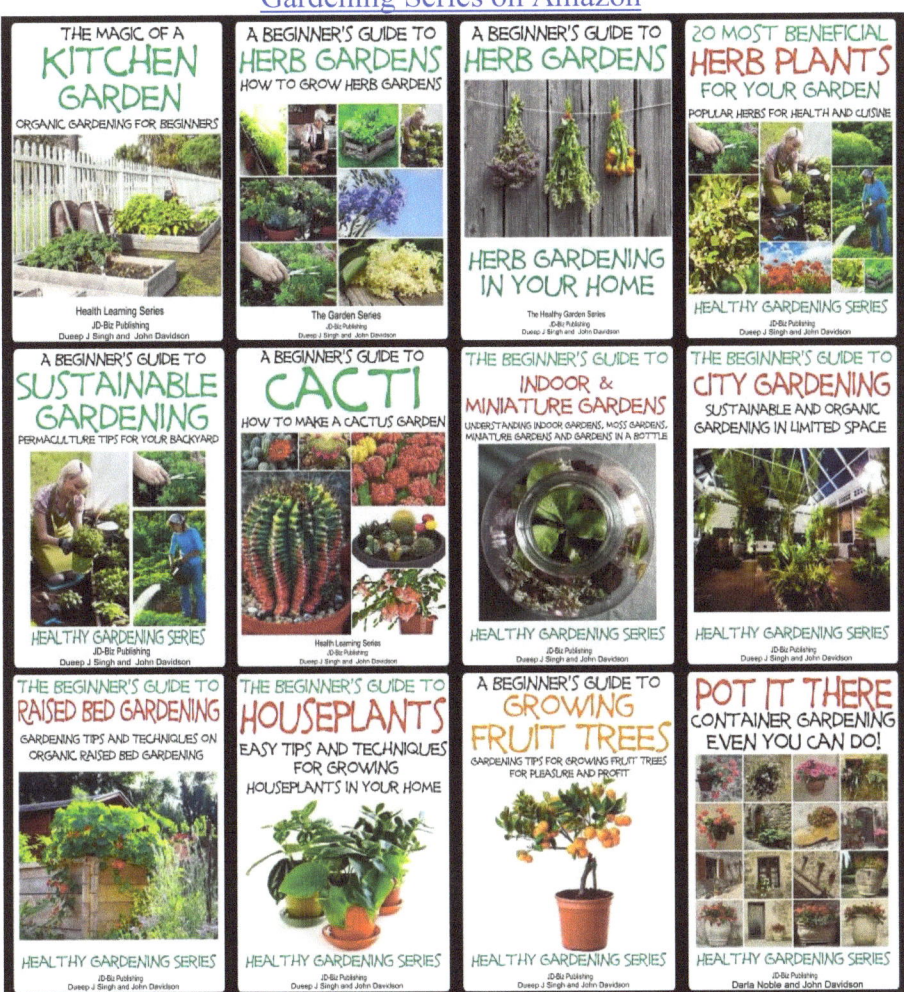

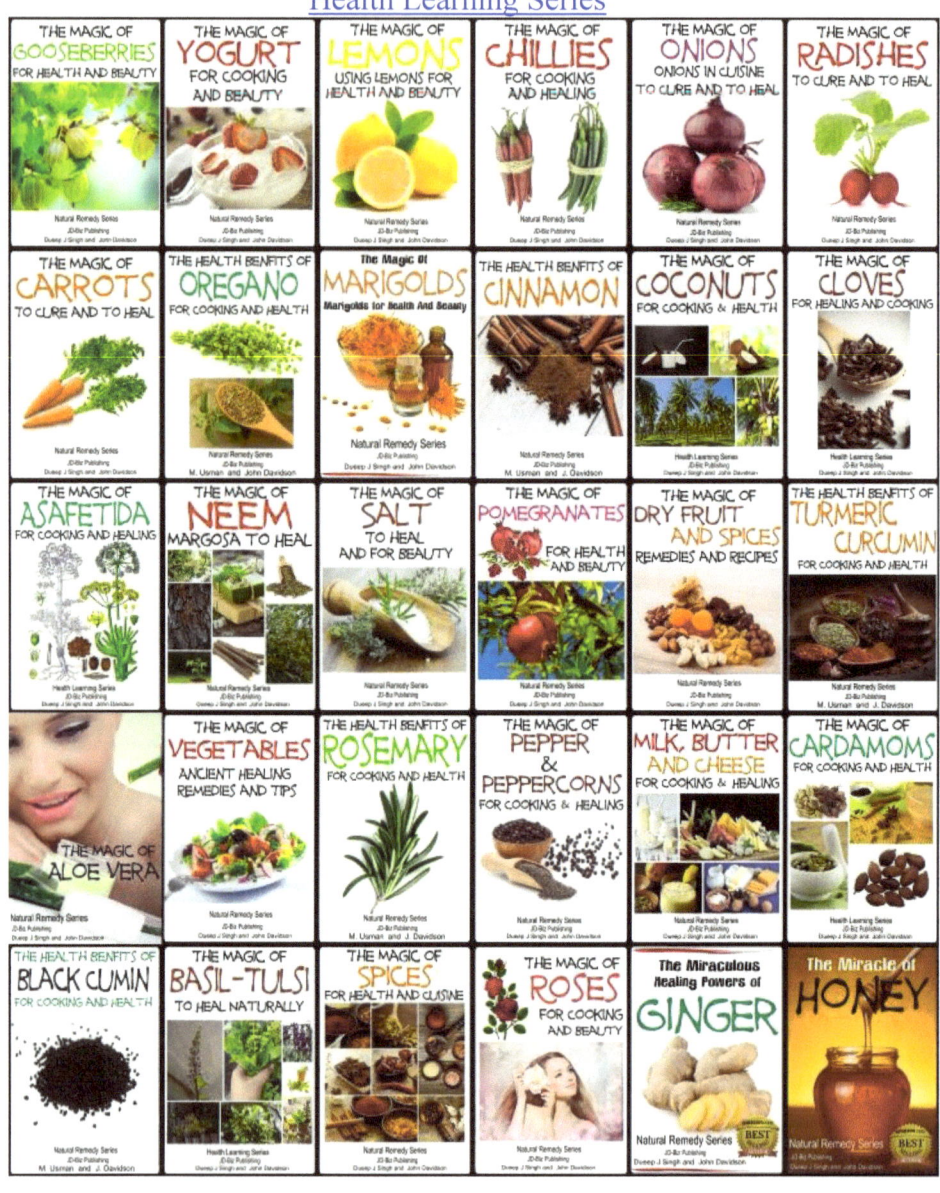

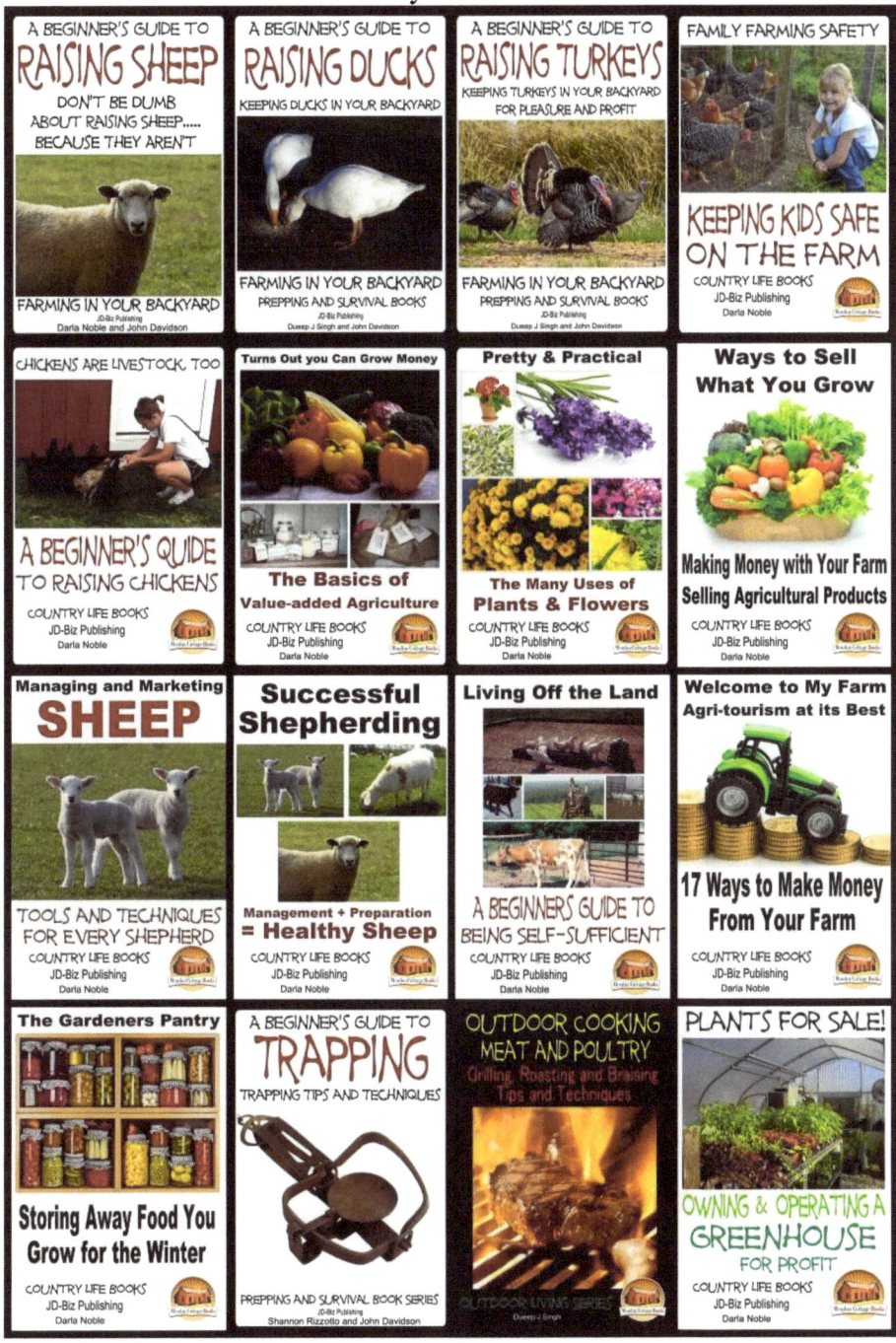

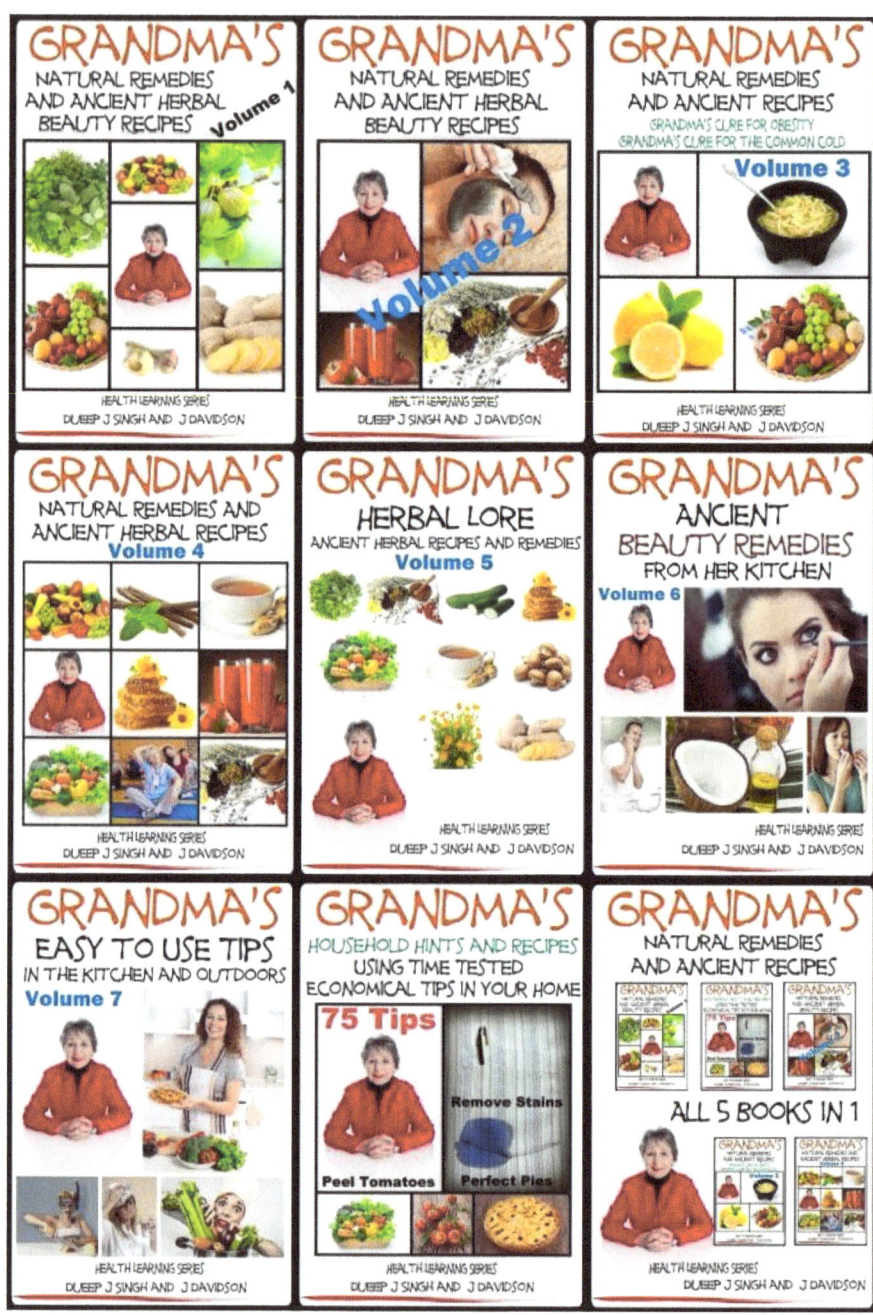

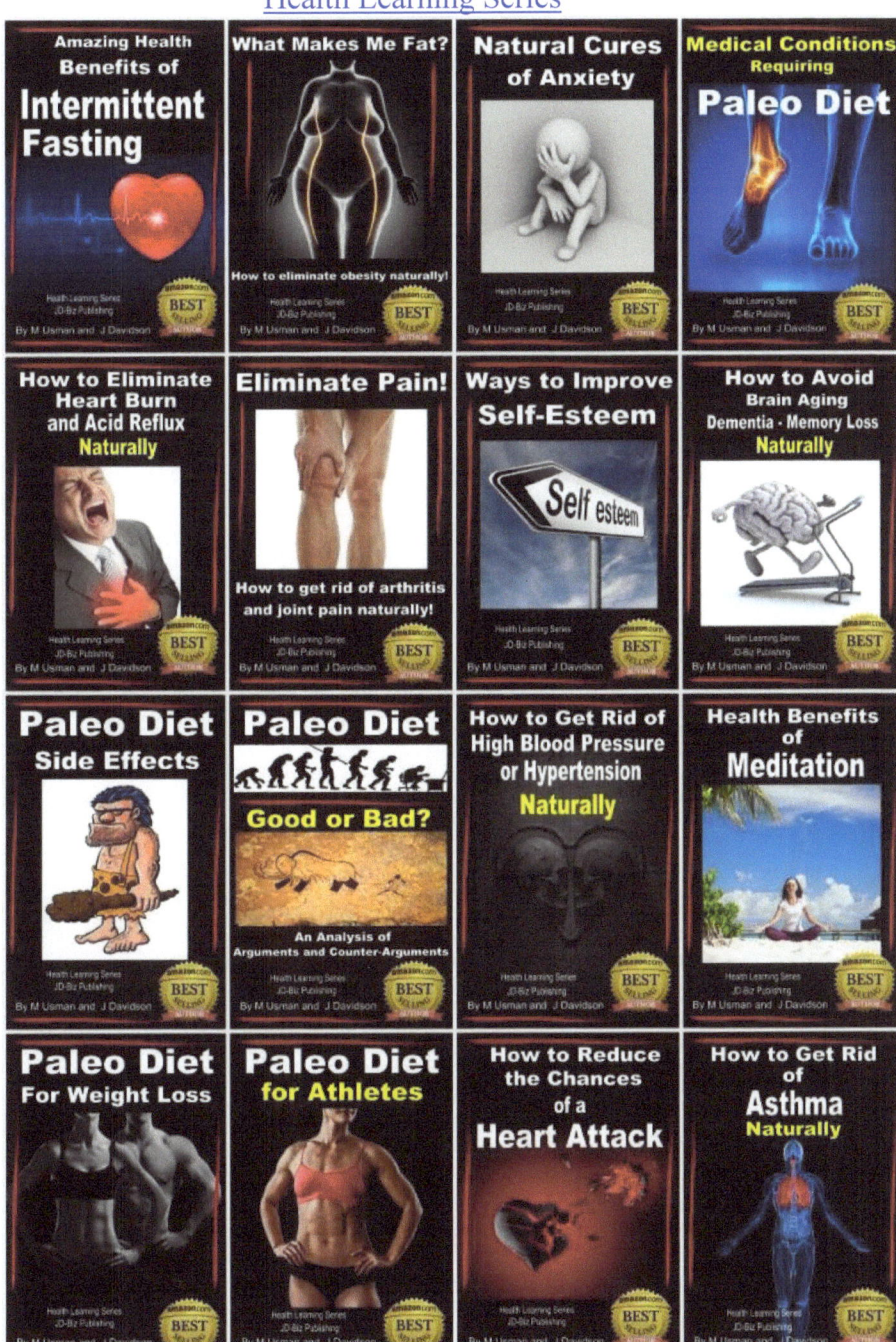

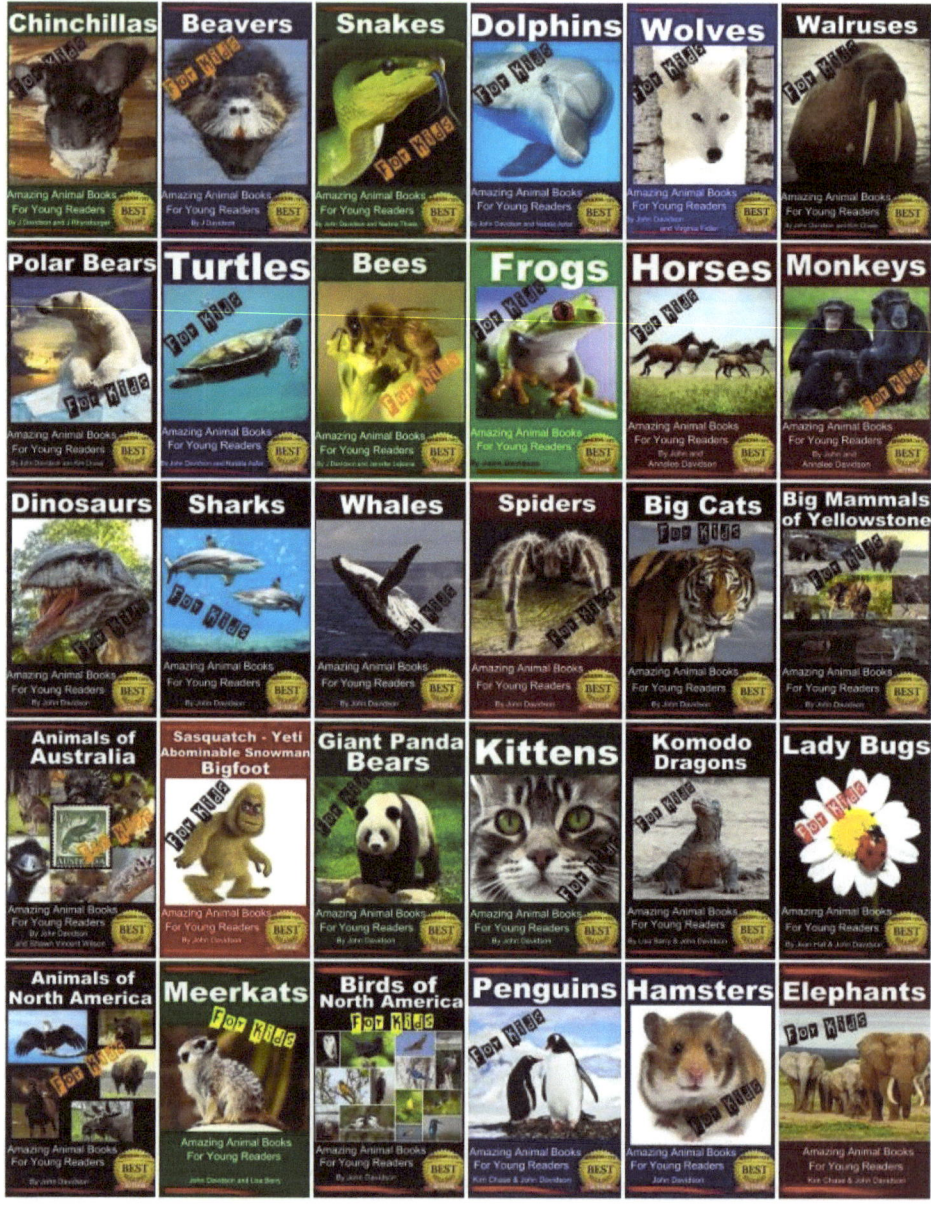

Learn To Draw Series

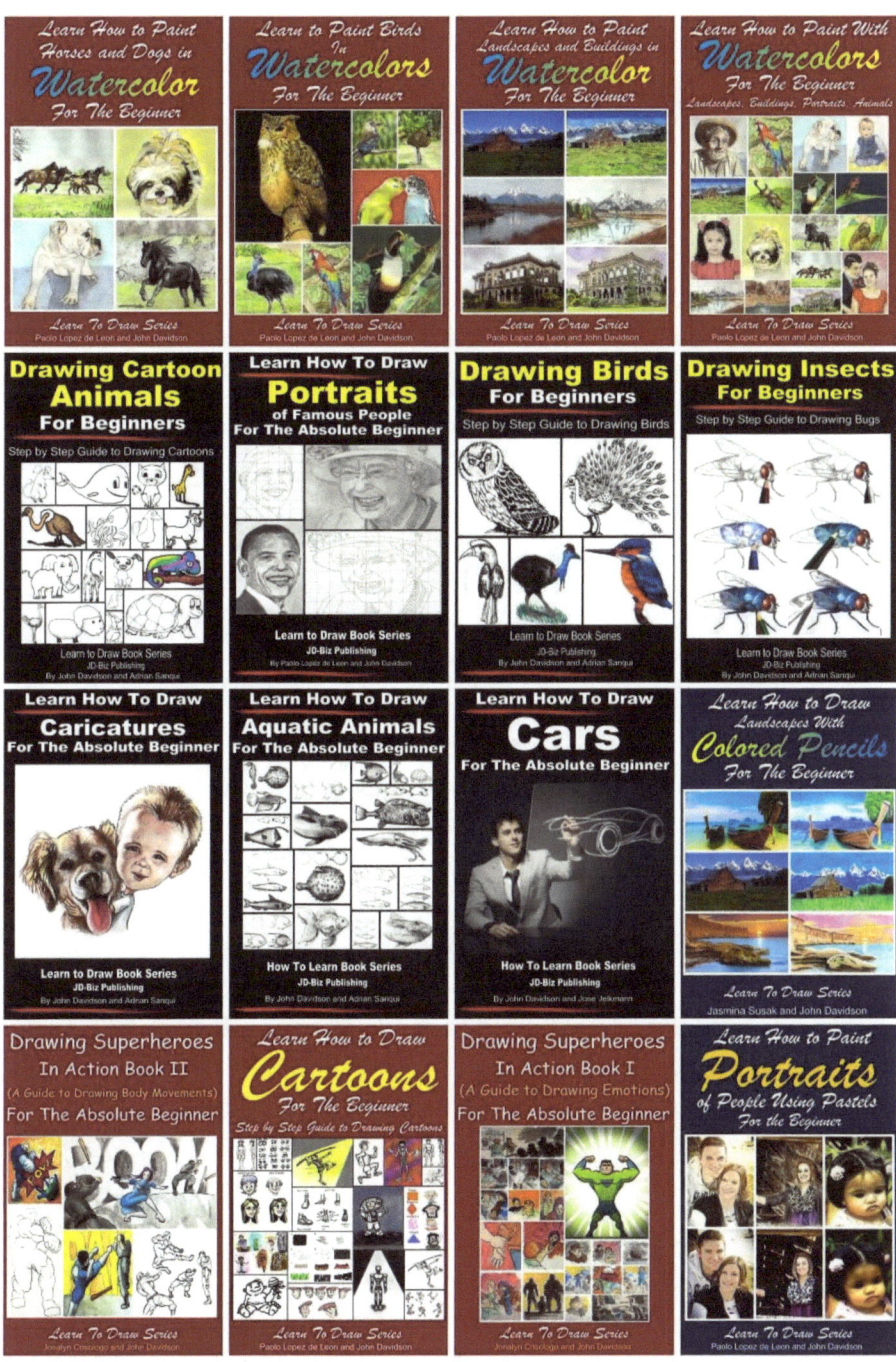

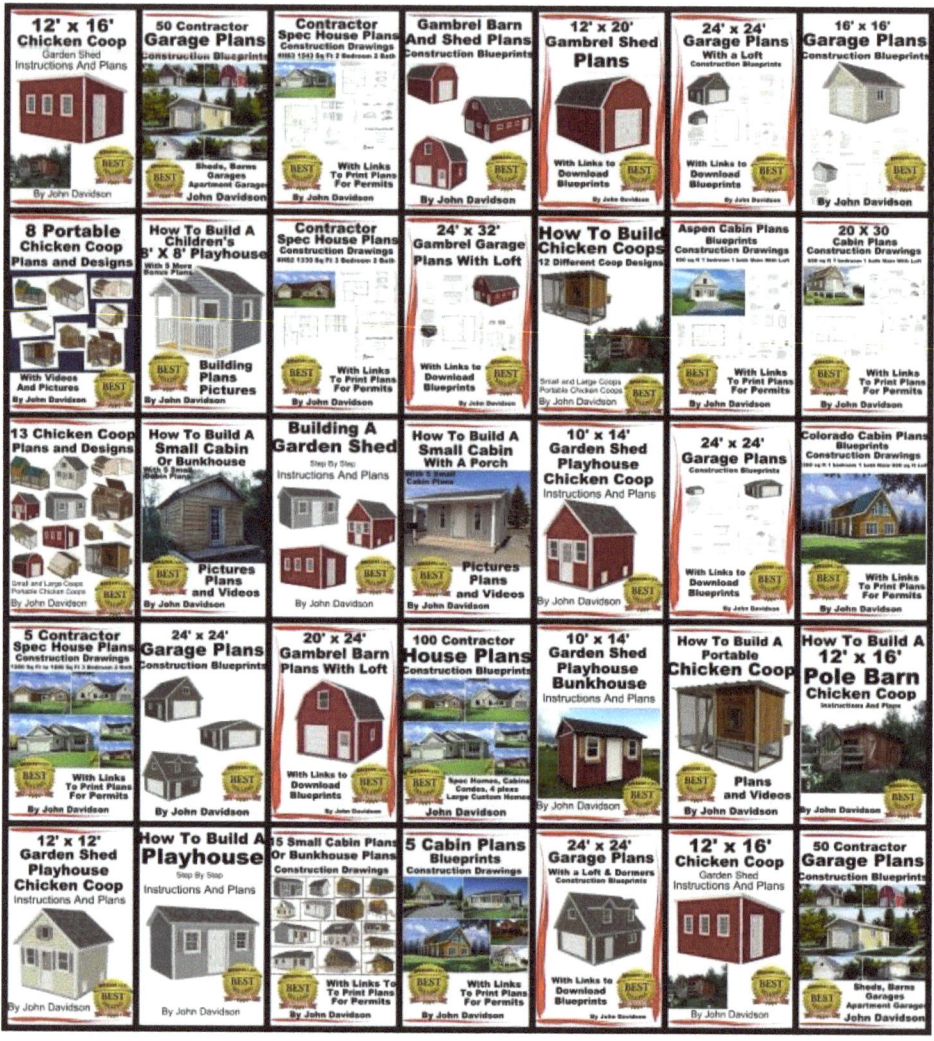

Entrepreneur Book Series

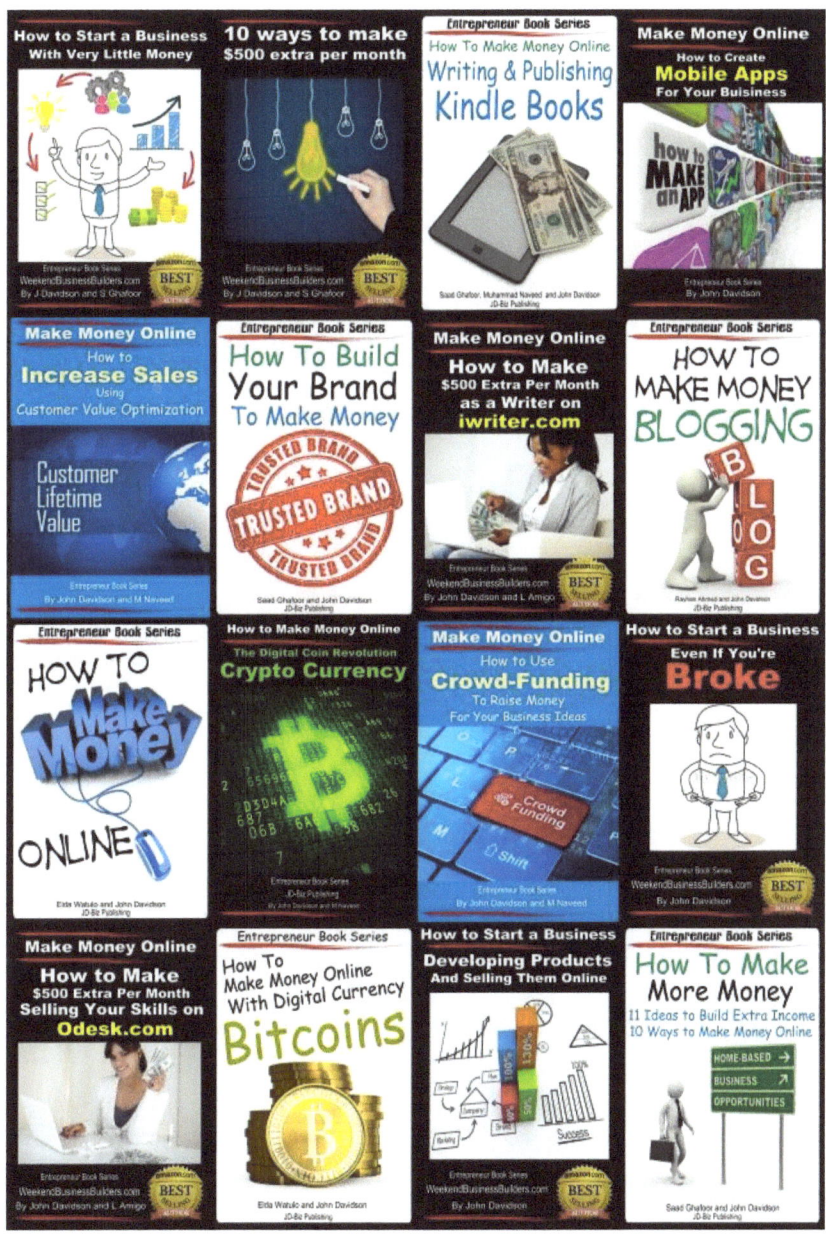

Our books are available at

1. Amazon.com

2. Barnes and Noble

3. Itunes

4. Kobo

5. Smashwords

6. Google Play Books

Download Free Books!

http://MendonCottageBooks.com

Publisher

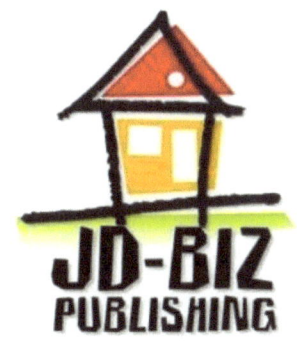

JD-Biz Corp

P O Box 374

Mendon, Utah 84325

http://www.jd-biz.com/

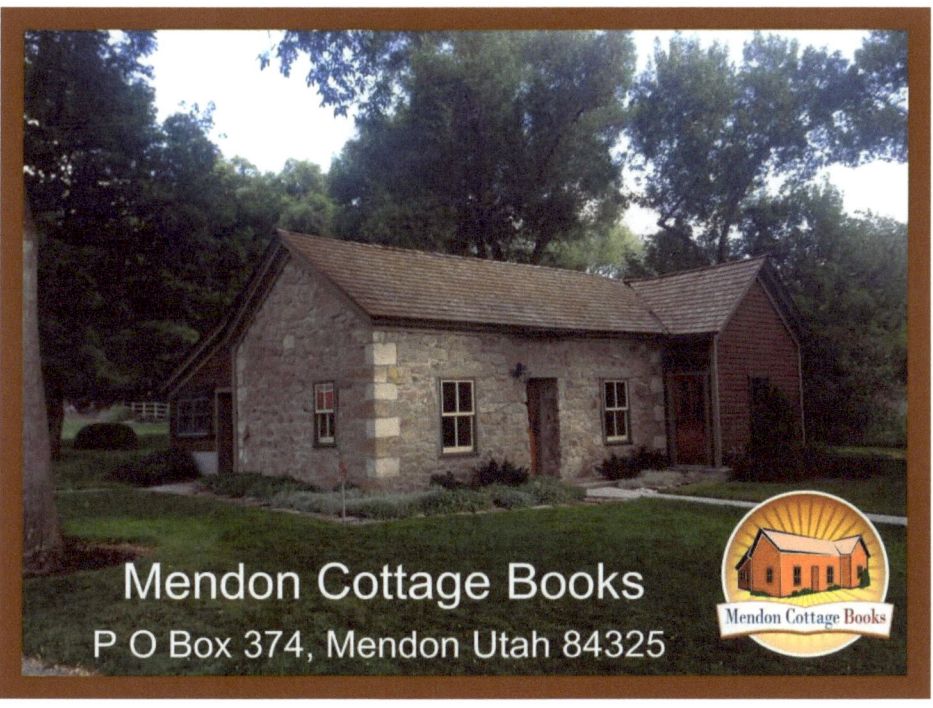

www.ingramcontent.com/pod-product-compliance
Lightning Source LLC
Chambersburg PA
CBHW040315010626
45792CB00022B/332